Spotlight on
Lab Assistants

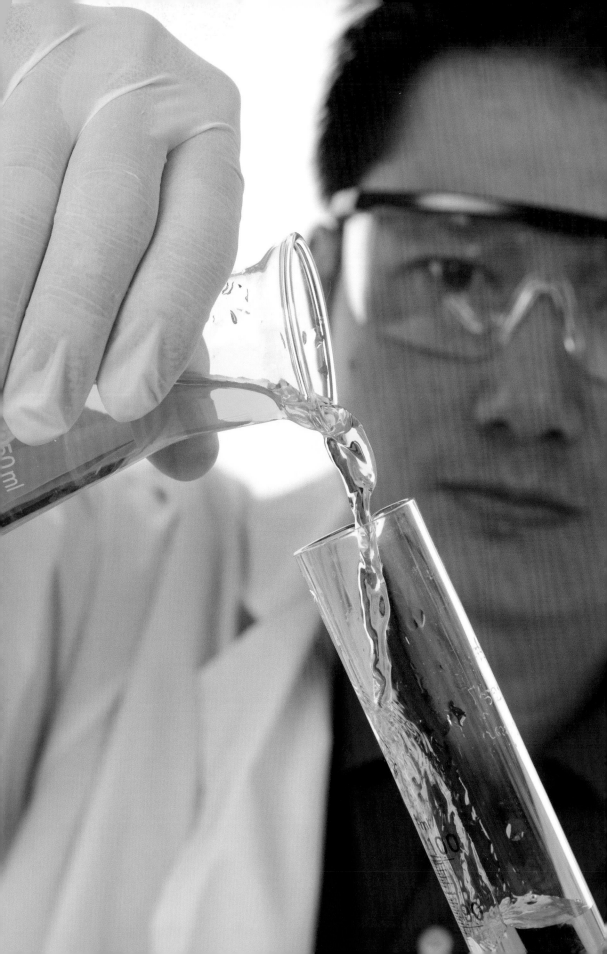

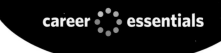
Spotlight on
Lab Assistants

Linda Kita-Bradley

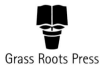

Grass Roots Press

Grass Roots Press thanks *DynaLIFE$_{Dx}$* and NAIT – The Northern
Alberta Institute of Technology for their valuable contributions to
Spotlight on Lab Assistants.

Grass Roots Press gratefully acknowledges the financial support
for its publishing programs provided by the following agencies:
the Government of Canada through the Canada Book Fund and
the Government of Alberta through
the Alberta Foundation for the Arts.
Alberta
Foundation
for the Arts

Library and Archives Canada Cataloguing in Publication

Kita-Bradley, Linda, 1958–, author
    Spotlight on lab assistants / Linda Kita-Bradley.

(Career essentials)
ISBN 978–1–77153–032–3 (bound)

    1. Medical laboratory assistants—Vocational guidance.
I. Title. II. Series: Kita-Bradley, Linda, 1958– Career essentials.

RB37.6.K58 2014   616.07'56023   C2013–906107–X

Printed and bound in Canada.

contents

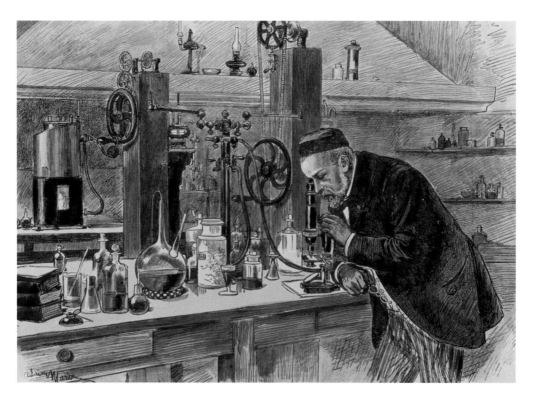

In the 1800s, doctors began to depend on instruments more than their powers of observation.

Introduction

Do you enjoy going for a blood test? Or a urine test? Or any kind of medical lab test? Not many people do. But lab tests help doctors diagnose, treat, and prevent disease.

Long ago, doctors did not rely on medical lab tests to diagnose disease. Instead, a doctor's diagnosis would depend on what they could observe with their eyes and hear with their ears. Making a diagnosis and treating illness was often hit or miss.

In the 1800s, doctors began to depend on instruments more than their powers of observation. The microscope became an important lab tool. By the mid-1800s, lab tests were being used to diagnose diseases such as **cholera** and **typhoid.**

Today, doctors and other health care professionals depend more on science to diagnose and treat illness. They depend on lab tests to analyze body fluids and samples of body parts such as hair, skin, and organs.

Medical lab assistants play a key role in health care. They support the work that is done in medical treatment and research. Lab assistants are part of a lab team, which is responsible for the quality of all lab tests.

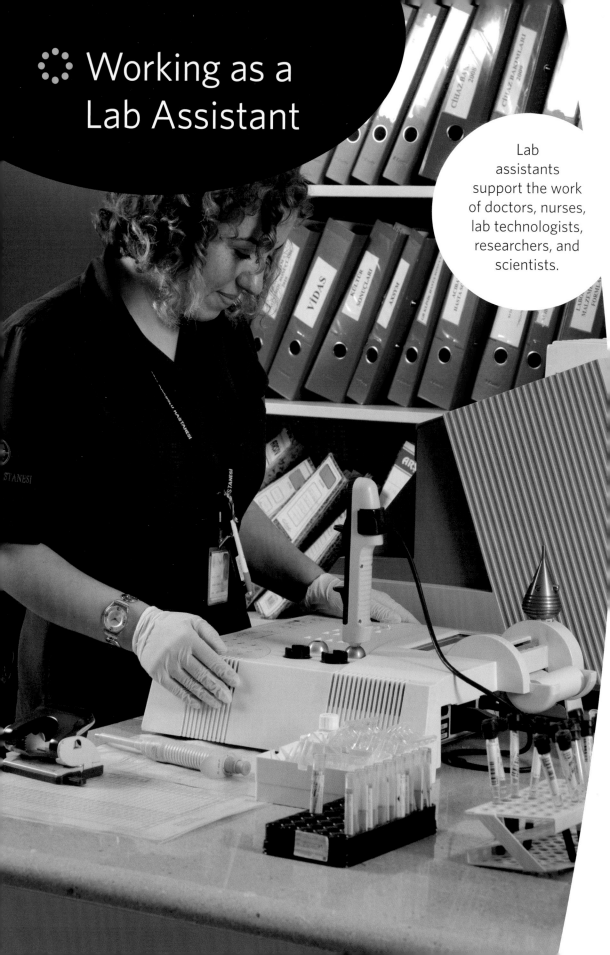

Working as a Lab Assistant

Lab assistants support the work of doctors, nurses, lab technologists, researchers, and scientists.

What does it take?

Imagine being a member of a team whose work makes a difference in people's lives. For example, the lab team helps doctors determine the correct diagnosis for patients. People's lives can depend on how well lab assistants perform their jobs.

Working in any area of health care takes passion and a specific set of skills. You will learn the skills in your training courses. If you have the passion, learning the skills will be that much easier.

Working as a lab assistant also takes a special kind of person. Read the list of statements. Do a lot of the statements describe you? If yes, you may have what it takes to be a medical lab assistant. With passion, the path to becoming a medical lab assistant will be an exciting one.

- I work well with others.
- I follow instructions well.
- I respect people's privacy.
- I work well independently.
- I can work under pressure.
- I have normal colour vision.
- I like working with equipment.
- I am good at solving problems.
- I like to pay attention to details.
- I communicate well with others.
- I can organize my time and tasks.
- I take pride in doing accurate work.
- I have good hand-eye coordination.
- I like to plan how I will approach a task.

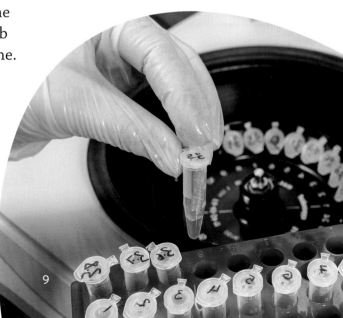

Lab assistants may work with different kinds of equipment.

What do lab assistants do?

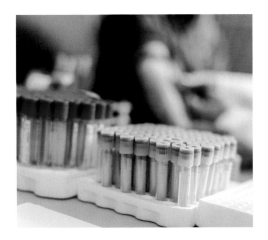

Lab assistants sort, label, and store samples.

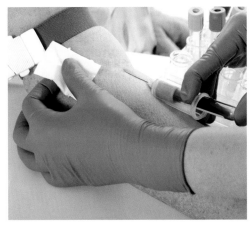

Lab assistants draw blood from veins.

Think about the last time you had to go for a blood test. Who took the sample of blood? Who made sure that your blood sample did not get mixed up with someone else's?

Lab assistants do many tasks that support the lab team and other health care professionals. Lab assistants collect and manage blood samples. They draw blood samples from veins. They sort, label, and store the samples. They prepare the samples for transport to other labs.

Lab assistants work with other kinds of samples as well. They explain to patients how to provide samples, such as **stool** samples.

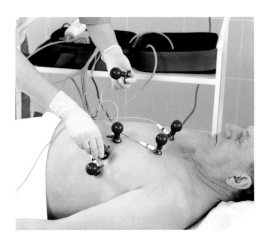

Some training programs teach lab assistants how to do an **ECG.**

Lab assistants may do some basic tests on urine samples. Samples of body fluids and solids are **biohazards**, so handling samples means following a lot of rules and regulations.

Lab assistants put specimens of blood on slides.

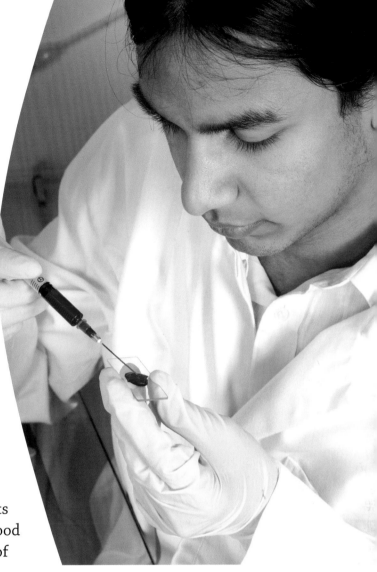

Lab assistants work with equipment. They load equipment with samples. For example, they put tubes of blood in centrifuges. A centrifuge separates **plasma** from the blood by spinning the blood at high speeds. Lab assistants also put **specimens** of blood on slides. The specimens of

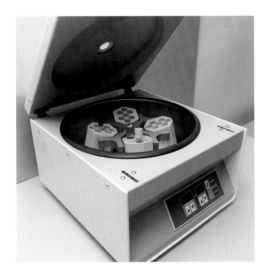

blood are then ready for the lab technologists to look at under a microscope. Lab assistants check lab equipment to make sure it is working. They may do small routine repairs on the equipment.

A centrifuge separates plasma from blood.

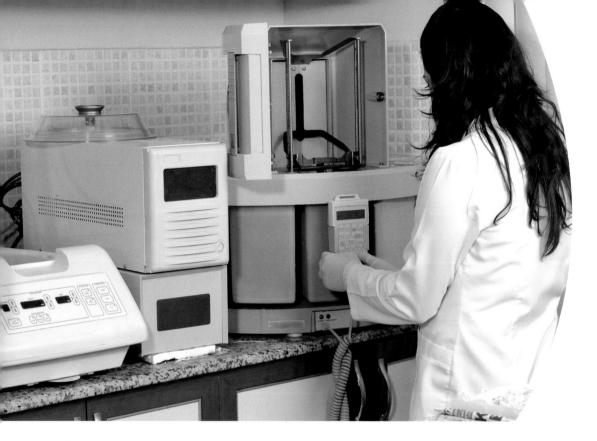

Labs have a lot of equipment.

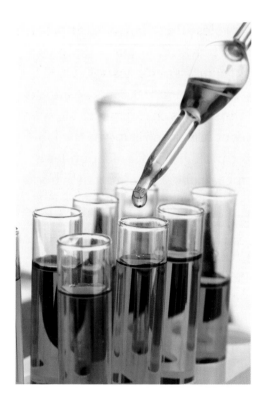

Lab assistants are also in charge of keeping labs clean and safe. They clean up after testing is done. They wash and sterilize glassware such as **flasks, beakers,** and **pipettes**. They also dispose of biohazardous waste such as samples and contaminated items like gloves.

Lab assistants sterilize glassware such as pipettes.

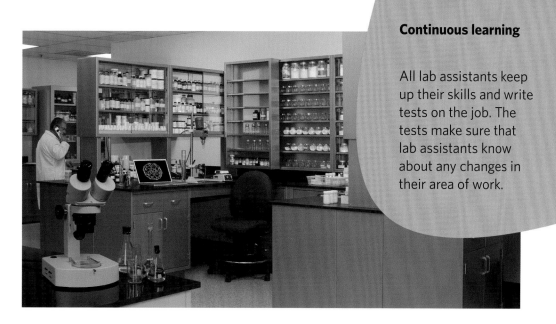

Continuous learning

All lab assistants keep up their skills and write tests on the job. The tests make sure that lab assistants know about any changes in their area of work.

Lab assistants may be responsible for stocking lab supplies.

Lab assistants support members of the lab team in other ways as well. They prepare and file documents. For example, they fill in claims for insurance companies. They may phone doctors with the results of patients' tests. Lab assistants may also be responsible for checking, ordering, and stocking lab supplies.

Many lab assistants specialize. Lab assistants specialize so they can do certain kinds of tasks. For example, some lab assistants specialize in working with **tissue** samples. Those lab assistants learn how to handle tissue samples and prepare them for testing. Other lab assistants work in specialized labs such as chemistry labs. Some work in **microbiology**.

In most cases, lab assistants do not work alone, especially when they start out. They often work on a team, and they work under the guidance of a lab manager or medical lab technologist. They can also get help from other lab assistants who are on the team and have experience.

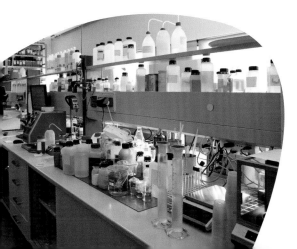

Some lab assistants work in chemistry labs.

Where do lab assistants work?

Medical settings

Lab assistants work in many different settings. Many work in medical settings such as clinics and hospitals. In both clinics and hospitals, lab assistants collect samples from people and they work in the lab.

Lab assistants who work in clinics spend a lot of time with clients. Clients go to clinics to have testing done. They take their test requisitions from their doctors with them. These requisitions list the samples that the lab assistant needs to collect.

People who go to clinics can be called patients or clients.

Lab assistants also carry out tasks such as getting samples ready for transport or restocking supplies. Some clinics send all their samples to a testing lab. Other clinics do some testing on site. If lab assistants work at clinics that do on-site testing, they carry out basic tests.

Test requisitions tell lab assistants what samples to collect.

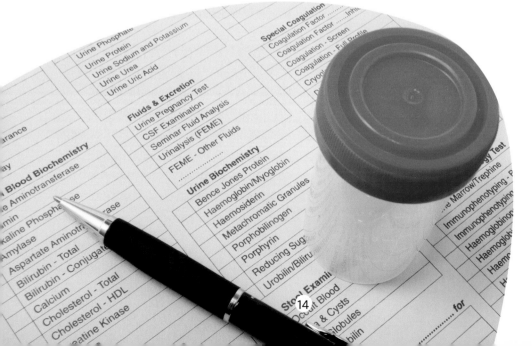

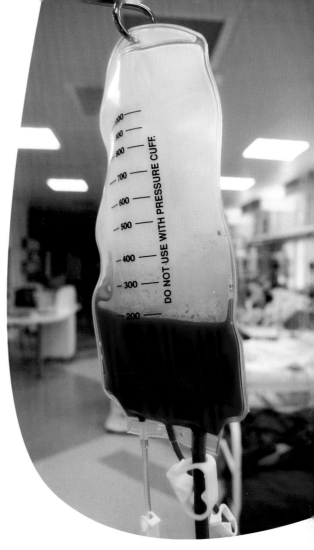

Some patients need blood transfusions. Lab assistants draw blood from those patients. The blood is tested for blood type and toxins.

DO NOT USE WITH PRESSURE CUFF.

Like in a clinic, lab assistants who work in hospitals spend a lot of time collecting samples. At the beginning of their shift, lab assistants receive collection lists. They go around to the hospital wards and collect samples from the patients on their lists. At any time, though, lab assistants who work in hospitals can be called to help deal with an emergency. In an emergency, lab assistants support the lab team by collecting blood samples.

Imagine nurses and doctors working madly to keep an accident victim alive. Imagine that at the same time, you are trying to insert a needle into the patient's vein. A road accident may mean that 20 people arrive in the hospital emergency at the same time. Some of those people may need **blood transfusions.**

Lab assistants must be ready to collect blood samples from injured people. The blood samples that lab assistants collect are tested for blood type and **toxins**. In emergency rooms, lab assistants do not work alone. A member of the health care team helps to keep patients calm so that lab assistants can collect the needed samples. Still, lab assistants must be able to stay focused under pressure. And they must have steady hands!

Ask the lab assistant

Joseph has worked in a clinic for two years. He says being a lab assistant is exciting because of the patient interaction.

Why did you become a lab assistant?

I had just graduated as a pharmacist back home and then my family came to Canada. To be a pharmacist in Canada, I would have to go back to university and do the pharmacy program again. So I thought I would try lab assistant, and it turned out great for me.

Describe a typical day at work in the clinic.

The morning is always the busiest part of the day. Sometimes I walk up to the back door when I'm getting to work and we haven't even opened up yet and I can see patients lined up for a block. So I know what I'm getting into that morning, and I really hope all my co-workers show up on time. We greet the clients. We put their personal information and test requisition details into the system. Then

"She said, 'If you didn't draw that blood that day, my dad could have died.' "

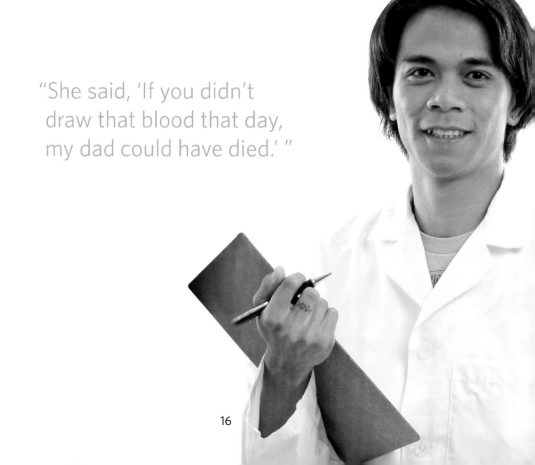

we follow what their test requisitions say. I look after patients from the start of the day to the end. It's like a cycle. When I'm done with one patient, I go on to the next one. That is the bulk of our work. Maybe 80 percent of our work is dealing with clients.

What do you do when you're not with clients?

We have what's called the backbench. This is where we process samples. We put samples in the centrifuge. We transfer urine samples into containers. We get samples ready for the couriers to take to base lab. Things like that. We used to do some testing, like pregnancy tests, but now we just do sugar testing. The other tests are done at our base lab. So you work as a team to get that extra stuff done, but you work as an individual with each patient.

How did you feel the first time you drew blood from a client?

Very nervous! You know, holding the needle, and my hand, when I'm nervous, shakes. The patients can see that you're shaking. Actually, for me it was nerve-wracking the very first time. My hands were sweating. I felt hot. I'm thinking, "Wow, this is for real. I really need to draw blood from a client." But after a couple of pokes, you gain your confidence.

Why do you use the word "poke"?

It's a gentle word. We use it all the time. Patients can visualize what we are going to do. If we say draw blood, they might not understand what we are going to do.

What do you find challenging as a lab assistant?

There are times I have to draw blood from babies. It's harder because they can't tell me what's going on. They just cry. And the mom is there, so that adds a lot of pressure. You really want to draw the blood in one poke. Make it work the first time.

What makes a good lab assistant?

Paying attention to detail. Accuracy. Checking doctors' medical codes, ordering the right tests, checking each requisition, making sure the doctor put the right patient labels on the right requisitions. You have to make sure you have the right patient sitting in the chair. You have to check IDs every time you see patients. You want to do everything right the first time. We're talking about people's health.

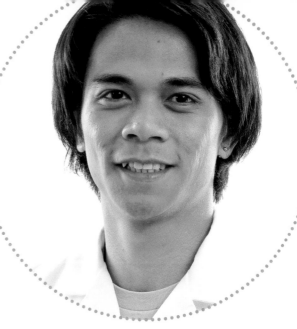

What makes you a good lab assistant?

I'm good at holding a lot of details in my head. Let's say, I call you in to take your blood and you're in the chair. Then I see a patient with a urine sample in their hand. They're wandering about because they forgot where to put the sample, so I have to help them out. At the same time, I have a patient in the ECG room removing their clothes for their test, and I've told them I'll be right back. In the meantime, all those other things are happening, but I have to remember that patient in the ECG room. She's there, waiting for the ECG test. She's going to miss me after a while.

Describe a memorable moment.

A daughter came in one afternoon with her father. They had a requisition for lots of tests to be done, and it's five minutes before closing time. But I took the dad in and collected everything and processed everything. Three days after, his daughter came back. And you know what she told us? She said, "If you didn't draw that blood that day, if you had turned us away because it was closing time, my dad could have died." That really touched me. Nothing can replace the gratefulness, the appreciation clients show for what you do.

What advice do you have about being a lab assistant?

We are dealing with the people's lives. We have a key role in the medical system, but sometimes we forget that. You know, the nurses, they're the ones that are in touch with the patient, directly helping the patient, and so sometimes the lab assistants are overlooked. So we have to remember what we do, the part we play.

Ask the lab assistant

Kelsey has worked in a hospital for eight years. She says being a lab assistant means making a lot of little decisions every day.

Why did you become a lab assistant?

One of my best friends had graduated from a lab assistant course and really loved what she was doing. I was doing vet medicine at the time and it wasn't going too well. I just wasn't very good at the animal practicum. I cried every day, just seeing the animals so sick or hurt.

So I tried lab assisting, and it's perfect for me. You get some patient contact, which I love. I couldn't be a nurse. That's too much patient contact for me. It's too personal.

Describe a typical day at work.

We collect a lot of blood! In the morning, first thing, we get our collection sheets. I usually have 20 to 30 patients to collect blood from. I collect the blood, then bring the samples down to the lab and get them ready for testing. The lab technologists do the testing and then the doctors who are in the hospital come down for the results, usually about noon. Most doctors get test results online. Some doctors phone in for results.

Do you do any testing on samples?

No. At this hospital, the lab technologists do all the testing. Our lab is set up to do about 40 different kinds of tests, and they're just the tests that are needed in emergencies, when the doctors need results right away. Any routine kinds of tests, we ship to a testing lab.

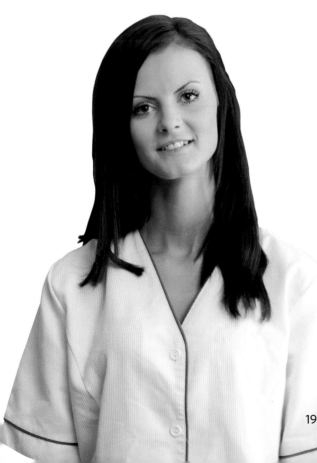

"'Oh, the vampire is here.' The patients love saying that."

Do you work in the same ward every day?

No. It's different every day. In the morning, I check the schedule. One day I might be on the maternity ward collecting blood from all the new moms. That's usually a pretty happy morning. The next day I might be assigned to the hospital's out-patient clinic, or I might be doing data entry in the lab most of the day, or working in emergency. So, yeah, every day is really different. Some days, I come in, blink, and the shift is over.

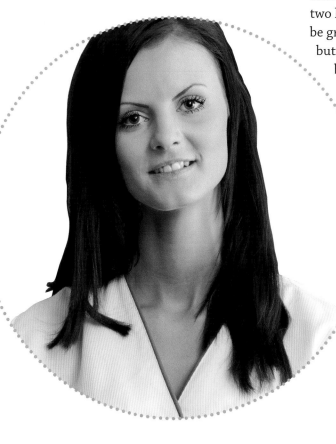

What do you do in the emergency room?

Collect blood. It's high stress. Everybody—the doctors, the nurses—are there waiting for you to collect the blood and the blood's not coming out of the person's vein. I mean some people come into emergency and they don't have a pulse! It's really hard to collect their blood. But the doctors are understanding. Sometimes you're there and a patient doesn't make it. The first time you see that, wow. You remember that.

How is working in a hospital different from working in a clinic?

At a clinic, people walk in on their own two legs. They're healthy. Some may be grumbly because they're fasting, but that's the worst you get. Drawing blood is easy because the people are healthy. They have better veins. Drawing blood is fast, like a two-minute interaction sometimes. But in a hospital, the patients are really sick. Some patients are unconscious; some have **dementia**. Sometimes the patient is curled on their side, maybe in pain, so you have to unfold their arm, talk to them, try to keep them as comfortable as you can. You're waking these people up a lot of the time.

How many lab assistants work each shift?

About 15 to 20. It depends. The mornings are always the busiest time, so there are always more of us working the morning shift. We have to cover all the wards and the emergency unit.

What is your favourite part of being a lab assistant?

Patient care for sure. You get patients in the hospital refusing to let you collect blood. You have to have that personality where you can approach patients and explain that collecting blood is for their own good, that it's their doctor's request. You have to be understanding, say "I'm really sorry to poke you this early in the morning." "Oh, the vampire is here." The patients love saying that.

What makes a good lab assistant?

You have to be compulsive about details. You always want to double-check everything. You always have to follow procedure. You have to be a rule follower. Patients remember the last time someone collected blood from them, and they always expect the same standards, the same procedure.

What advice do you have about being a lab assistant?

Try it. It's one of those jobs that suits a lot of different kinds of people. You can do so many different kinds of things. Really, there is a position in lab assisting for everyone.

Diagnostic and testing labs

diagnostic: helping to identify illness or disease

Labs cost a lot of money to build and run, so many clinics do not have their own labs. Those clinics send their samples to diagnostic and testing labs. Some diagnostic and testing labs receive thousands of samples every day from clinics, hospitals, and health care professionals.

Lab assistants who work in diagnostic and testing labs do not work with clients. The main part of their work is managing samples and processing test requisitions. They also prepare samples for testing.

Lab assistants in testing labs need to be able to organize their workloads. Sometimes doctors need test results right away. Those tests are high priority. Lab assistants need to recognize when tests are high priority. They need to prepare the samples quickly so that the lab technologists can begin testing. Organizing workloads means knowing which tasks must be done right away and which tasks can wait until later.

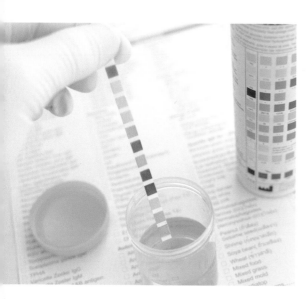

Lab assistants carry out basic tests on urine samples.

Research labs

Lab assistants may work part-time on special projects in a research lab. Some research projects run human trials—testing new drugs on humans. Human trials may require taking blood samples from people.

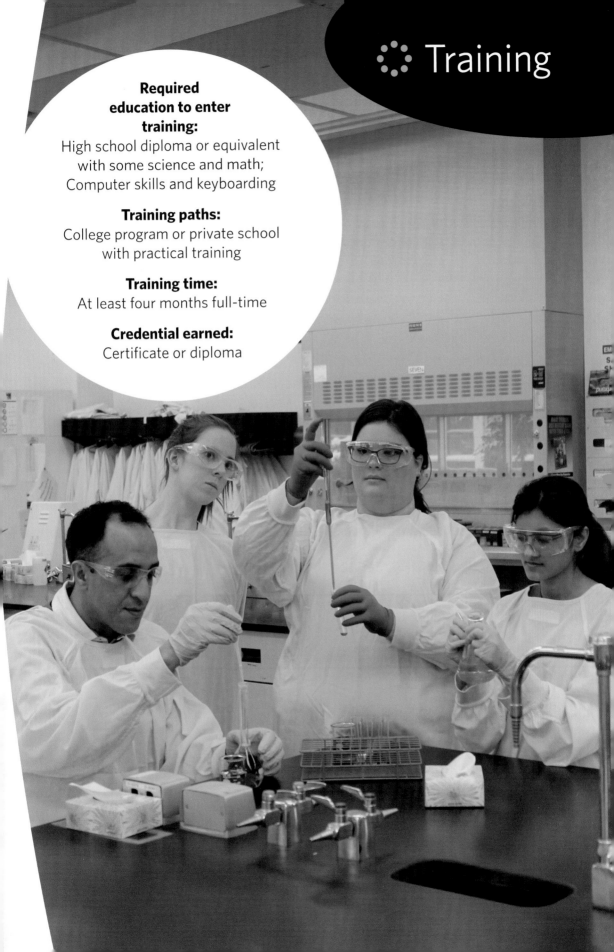

Required education to enter training:
High school diploma or equivalent with some science and math; Computer skills and keyboarding

Training paths:
College program or private school with practical training

Training time:
At least four months full-time

Credential earned:
Certificate or diploma

Training

What does *bio* mean in the word *biology*? Where does **saliva** come from? What makes cuts stop bleeding? Did you know that your heart beats 100,000 times a day?

Training to be a lab assistant includes learning about the body—the structure of the body and how the body works. But learning about the human body is just the start.

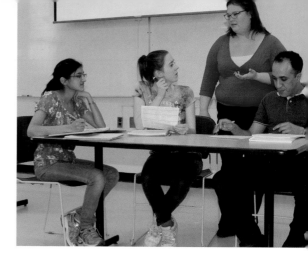

Students discuss ideas and ask questions in class.

What to expect

Training courses for lab assistants have something for everyone. They offer a balance between class time and practical time.

Class time

In class, instructors give lectures on the information that lab assistants need to know. Many instructors come to class with years of experience working in labs or health care. Students have a chance to discuss ideas with their instructors. They have a chance to ask questions about what they read in their textbooks.

Instructors also set up learning opportunities for the students. For example, students do research, make group presentations, watch training videos, and work on individual projects.

What do lab assistants learn about in class?

- medical language and how to understand it
- bones, tissue, organs, cells, and body fluids like urine and saliva
- the systems of the body and how they work, like how blood flows through the body
- the systems of the body and diseases
- basic math used in the lab
- using lab documents
- working in a safe and healthy way
- communicating with other health care professionals
- dealing with conflict on the job
- the ethics and laws that relate to working in a lab

24

Lab time

Lab time means hands-on time. Lab time gives students the chance to use and apply what they learn in class. For example, in class students learn about blood and what it is made of. They learn how blood flows through the body. During lab time, students spin tubes of blood in a centrifuge. They see how the plasma separates from the blood. Students also practise collecting blood samples.

During lab time, instructors offer a safe, caring place where students can develop their skills. Students practise the procedures that they will carry out in the workplace. Instructors observe the students closely. They help the students with their technique. They give the students feedback.

What do lab assistants practise during lab time?

- hygiene, like handwashing
- collecting blood samples
- using sample-collecting kits
- labelling, sorting, and packing samples
- using lab equipment
- doing basic tests on samples
- communicating with patients and clients

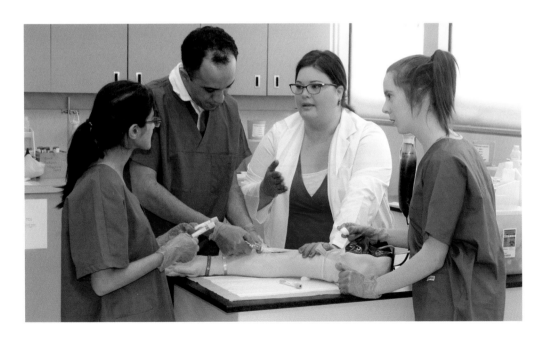

In lab, students practise how to draw blood.

Practicum

Lab assistant programs often include a practicum. In a practicum, students join a lab team at a workplace. The practicum can last one week, a few weeks, or longer. The length of the practicum depends on the length of the training program.

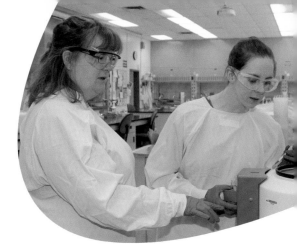

Staff at the workplace support students on practicum.

Become a specialist

Lab assistants can specialize in many different areas. They learn how to prepare samples for the lab technologists in one or more of these areas:

- **Biochemistry**
  Studying chemical reactions in the body

- **Cytology**
  Studying cells in the body

- **Histology**
  Cutting and staining tissue

- **Histopathology**
  Examining tissue that is diseased

- **Immunology**
  Studying the immune system

- **Microbiology**
  Studying small organisms, such as bacteria and viruses

Lab assistants who specialize get on-the-job training. Some training programs teach lab assistants to work in all the different areas.

During practicum, students observe members of a lab team at work. Students learn to do basic tasks in the lab. They learn to work with clients and patients. Staff at the workplace and members of the lab team supervise the students. Students are rarely, if ever, left to work on their own.

The practicum helps students learn what it means to be a lab assistant. Students face the challenges that they will deal with when they start working in the lab. They develop their skills, and they gain confidence in their work.

The practicum also helps students get an idea of what kind of lab they would like to work in. For example, some students enjoy lab work more than interacting with patients and clients. Those students might decide to look for a job in a testing lab.

Ask the instructor

Jackie teaches in a full-time lab assistant program at a college. She works in the lab with students. She teaches students about the different kinds of lab work that they will do in each area of the lab.

What helps students have success in their training?

Being organized. How are they going to deal with five courses at one time? How are they going to organize their family time, work time, and study time? How are they going to organize all the books they have to bring to school every day? One student told me she felt like she was carrying four bags of groceries and things were starting to fall out of the bags. I gave her some hints about how to organize her notes, her time. Things went better for her after that.

What kinds of things do students do in class?

There's a lot less of the teacher as a "sage on the stage" going on. We get the students to be more active, doing things like research and discussion. We ask for a lot of group work, which is good, because the job itself is about being part of a team. The soft skills are really important. I mean working as a team, communication, being professional, understanding others, getting along with others, having patience. You can learn the technical skills of the job, but lasting in this career means mastering those soft skills.

"When a student's interest peaks, that's it! Don't bother paying me, 'cause seeing that interest is pay enough."

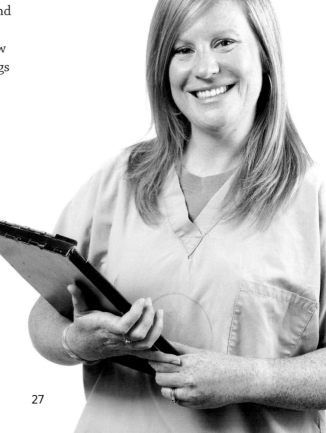

What skills help a student succeed in a lab assistant program?

- Basic math skills
- Basic computer skills
- Being able to recognize the key information in reading material
- Being able to take notes in class and organize them
- Being able to organize family, work, and study time
- Being able to apply the soft skills, such as getting along with others

What computer skills do students need?

To get into our program, students have to be able to keyboard 30 words a minute with 90 percent accuracy. They have to feel comfortable with computers. They need to be familiar with common software like Word and PowerPoint. They learn how to do data entry, order tests, and enter patient information into a program. They need to use e-mail. Some assessments are done online.

Do students need math?

They need to have some math skills. For example, they need to be able to do calculations with percents and volume. If I give you 100 percent bleach and tell you I need a 10 percent solution, you need to know how to make that solution.

What kinds of reading and writing do students do?

They have to do a lot of reading before classes. They get reading materials that help them prepare for class. I would say, on average, students have between two and three hours of homework a night—reviewing notes, reading and making notes, studying. Reading is the biggest part of homework. The key thing is knowing how to get the important information out of the reading material.

Writing is mostly note-taking. But they also have to write their assignments and summarize the steps they need to do for work in the lab.

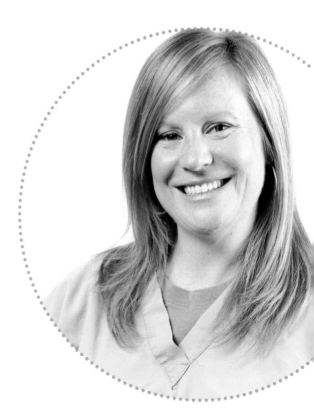

How are students assessed?

They have theory exams and hands-on exams. Each is worth about 50 percent of the final mark. There are a lot of little assessments throughout the course, not just one large exam at the end. Students have to pass all of their courses to be able to go on their practicum.

What challenges do students face?

Some students don't have faith in themselves. That's challenging for sure. They think they don't have what it takes, but they do. It takes them time to figure out they can do the course, to gain confidence in themselves.

What do you enjoy most about teaching?

For me, it's seeing the students develop. I love seeing them doing their practicum. They're so professional. It's sending them out there and seeing the change in them. The best part is seeing them get interested in something that they could do as a life's work. When a student's interest peaks, that's it! Don't bother paying me, 'cause seeing that interest is pay enough, right?

How do students stay motivated?

We give the students the meat and potatoes of the big subjects. The course time is so limited that we have to get right into things. The students love that. They're so interested they just want to learn more. And the students become good friends. They motivate each other. Marks are a big motivator too, right? The students want to do well.

What advice do you have about training as a lab assistant?

There's something about the lab that drew each student into the program. So many things they learn really grab their attention. That interest becomes multiplied a hundred times once students start the program.

Thinking about starting a training program?

Do you have enough time?

Training programs offer courses full-time, part-time, online, or through distance education. All of these options demand a commitment of time. In addition to time spent in class, you have to consider study time, travel time, and time spent in practicum.

Do you have enough money?

The costs of training programs add up quickly. You need to think about the cost of courses, textbooks, equipment, and

Before you train

Most programs require that students get a police security check before they start training.

travel. Career counsellors can help you find funds to support your training. For example, they can help you find and apply for a student loan from the government.

Do you need child care?

Training courses may be scheduled for weekdays, evenings, or weekends. Talk to friends and family, and check out child care programs in your community. Sorting out child care before enrolling in a training course will reduce stress later on.

Making the decision to train for a new career is exciting, but it can also be life-changing. Such a decision cannot be made lightly. Training takes planning, time, money, and a lot of hard work.

At the same time, training for a new career opens doors to new opportunities, new people, and new ways of thinking.

What should you look for in a medical lab assistant program?

- Does the program have a good reputation?

- Does the program follow rules set by the government?

- Are the instructors experts in the subjects they teach?

- What are the school's facilities like?

- How much time is spent on hands-on training?

- What kinds of support does the school offer to students?

Ask the student

Colleen started training as a lab assistant right after she graduated from high school. She says her training experience has been informative.

Why did you decide to train as a lab assistant?

I love biology and I wanted to do something in the health field. I thought it would be a good place to start because I can expand from here later on if I want.

How did you prepare for the training?

I moved across the country for one thing. My aunt and uncle offered to let me live with them while I was at school. This is my first time living away from my family. It was a big adjustment all at once. My friends aren't here, so I don't have much of a social life. But that's good in a way. Fewer distractions.

What are you learning?

Tons of stuff. Urine analysis, blood collection, microbiology. We're kind of like the hired hands in the lab. We learn to do all the prep work for testing, but we're also given the knowledge of what's behind what we do and why we do it. So this means we won't be just blindly following instructions on the job.

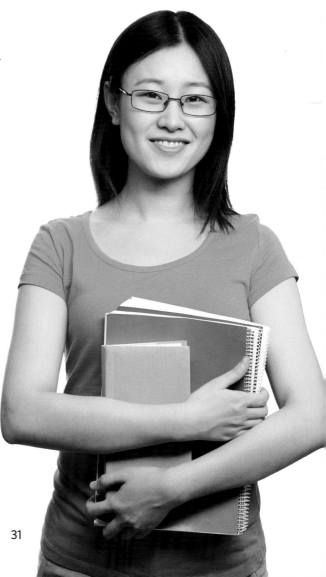

"I don't feel like anyone's trying to get a better grade than everyone else. We all want each other to succeed."

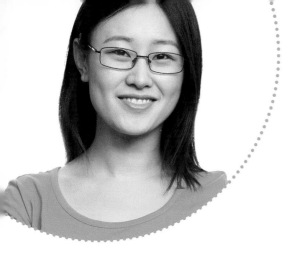

What is your favourite part of the course?

I like looking through the microscope. We're into hematology now so we're looking at the blood, the blood cells, and how they tell you so much about the body. That's just fascinating to me.

What do you find challenging about the training?

The workload can get heavy at times. This week we have three tests and two assignments and there's a lot of information to know for one test. So I continuously have to review and go over things, which can be tiring. I guess the hardest part is when all the tests come in the same week.

How do you cope with all the information you have to learn?

Asking questions is really important. If you don't know, ask. The instructors are always ready to answer questions. And cue cards. They've helped me a lot. Just writing things out on the cards helps me remember. And reviewing each night helps, instead of trying to cram for a test the night before.

How did you feel during the first few days of training?

When I walked down the hallway the first day, all the other students were just standing around, waiting to go into the classroom. Everyone's eyeballing each other, trying to figure out what everyone's story is. I talked to the girl sitting behind me in class. We ate lunch together. And as the days went by, we all became a big team.

How do the students work as a team?

When one of us is going through a hard time, say with blood collection, we're all really supportive. I don't feel like anyone's trying to get a better grade than everyone else. It's not cutthroat. We all want each other to succeed.

Is the training what you expected?

We look back at the textbooks and see what we've covered so far. It's crazy. To take all of this in and then remember it! We're surprised at ourselves. We're impressed that we can do it. You don't think you can do it when you look at the textbook on the first day. You think, how am I going to do this?

What advice do you have about training to be a lab assistant?

Make sure you're not queasy. Make sure you can handle blood and body fluids. Make sure you have an interest in biology and health, because that will definitely help. And make sure you know how to manage your time.

Ask the student

Malika is in a full-time training program at a college. She is married with two young children. She says that her training experience has been excellent.

Why did you decide to train as a lab assistant?

I was studying in a medical program back home. When we came to Canada, I wanted to continue studying, but I had to work while my husband got his vet's licence. I worked in a daycare, but I really wanted to work in health. Now my husband is working as a vet and my kids are older, so I can study. I want to do it for me. I didn't do any upgrading, so I decided that I would take a short course like lab assisting to see how things went.

How did you prepare for the training program?

I was frustrated because I had to leave my husband. We live in a small town. My husband stayed there to work. I came here to the city with my two kids and rented an apartment. My sister lives here and has her own family, but she helped me a lot. She helped me find a really good babysitter for my daughter. And I had to find a place for my son in school. He's six years old.

How do you balance looking after your kids and studying?

My kids are very good. When they are together, they play. When I'm doing homework, my son sits beside me and he

"The first week of training, I can tell you, I felt a little scared. It's different here in Canada."

brings a book and he sits with me. They go to sleep at 9:00 and after that, I have time to concentrate. I have about three or four hours of homework every night. Not always, but definitely when there is an exam coming up. My husband comes here on the weekends. If I have an exam, my sister will take the kids for me so I can study.

How did you feel during the first few days of training?

The first week of training, I can tell you, I felt a little scared. It's different here in Canada. Back home, we get more theory. We listen a lot. But here, it's more practical. I got my first lab assignment and I didn't know how I was going to do it. But I did it. And when I compare that first assignment with my assignments now, I think, oh my gosh, I didn't know anything when I started.

What do you find challenging about the course?

English is my second language. Sometimes in class, the instructor will ask a question. I know the answer but I don't raise my hand because I'm afraid

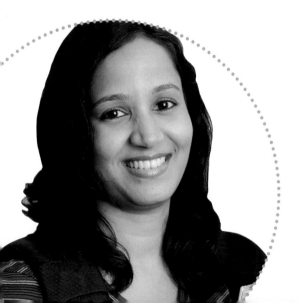

I won't say things right. And in the beginning, I had some difficulty with listening, understanding. But I'm getting better, more confident.

What is your favourite part of the course?

The labs. We do things with our hands, so we actually experience the things we have to do. So if I make a mistake, I know, oh okay, I won't make that mistake again. You learn from your mistakes.

What keeps you motivated?

My husband is very supportive. He tells me, you can do it. And he really helps me now. Before, when I wasn't training and he was working, I had to do everything. He came home from work and he did nothing. But now on the weekends, he tells me, you go and study. And he takes the kids. He's learning to cook and clean. I told him not to forget these things when I move back home!

What kind of lab assisting job do you hope to get?

I want to work in the out-patient lab at the hospital in my town. I'm excited about working with the different kinds of people, patients, who come to the lab.

What advice do you have about training to be a lab assistant?

I'd say go for it, because it's a short course and you learn so many interesting things.

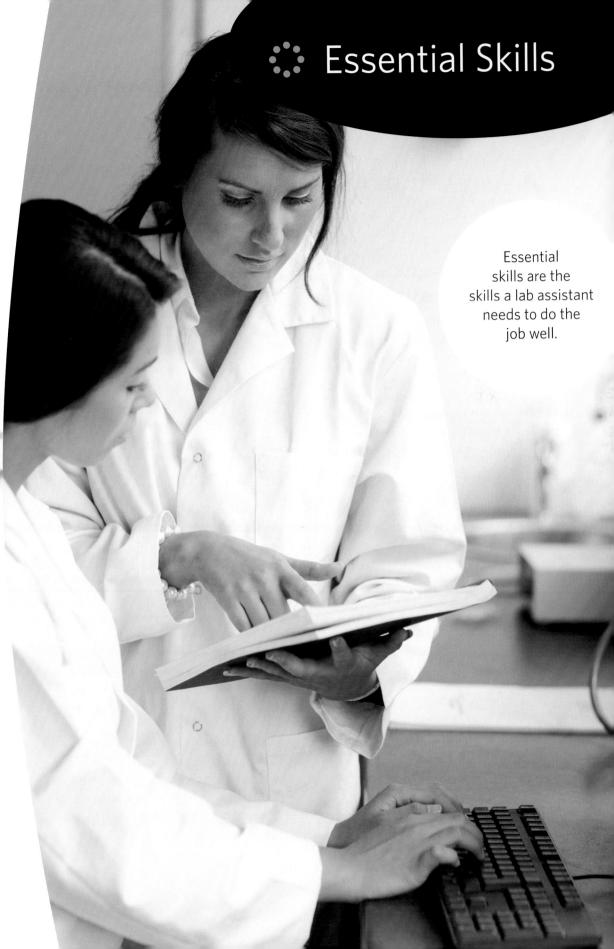

Essential skills are the skills a lab assistant needs to do the job well.

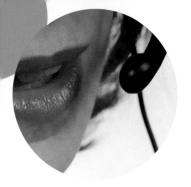

Meet Eva

Eva has been a lab assistant for ten years in a big city hospital. Eva's stories will show which essential skills are important in her work, and why.

Read Eva's first story to find out what she learned about communication early in her career.

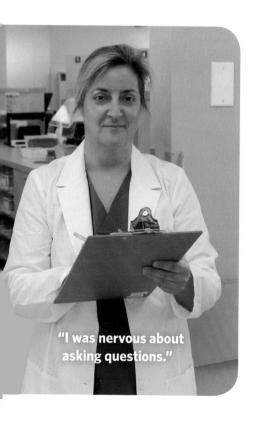

"I was nervous about asking questions."

Eva's story

Right after graduation, I was hired on as a lab assistant at this hospital. Everyone I worked with was great. They were ready to help me out at any time, but still, for some reason, I was nervous about asking questions. I felt, "Hey, I just graduated, so I should know everything."

My main job is collecting blood. I started collecting blood from patients on my very first day of work. Things were going okay. Then I had a bit of trouble with one patient. I couldn't find his vein. I asked a co-worker to help. She told me to turn the patient's wrist a little to move the tendon out of the way. It worked! Then wouldn't you know it, I walked into the next room and the patient wasn't in her bed. She was sitting on her chair flipping through a magazine. I didn't know whether I should ask her to lie down on the bed before I collected her blood. I wondered—is it better if she is lying down?

I really didn't want to ask my co-worker for advice again. I was afraid she'd think I couldn't do my job. I didn't want to be that person who asked, you know, the stupid question. But I wanted to make sure the patient was comfortable while I was collecting her blood. So I asked. I didn't want to risk harming the patient in any way.

And here it is ten years later and I'm still asking questions. Things change so fast—technology, the way we do things, everything. I just have to accept the fact that I will never know everything there is to know in this job. I just have to keep on learning and asking questions.

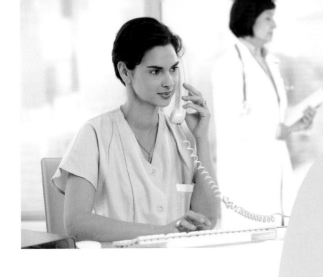

Communication also means having good listening skills.

A key essential skill that lab assistants need is oral communication. Lab assistants communicate with many people in a day. For example, they communicate with co-workers. They communicate with health care professionals such as doctors and nurses, and they communicate with patients.

Eva learned early in her career that asking questions is an important part of communication. The work that lab assistants do affects people's health, so lab assistants must be 100 percent sure that they do their work accurately.

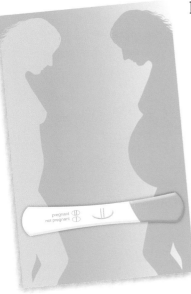

Lab assistants use diagrams to help patients understand instructions.

All in a day's work

- Eva has to collect blood from a patient who is nervous. Eva asks the patient why he is nervous. Talking relaxes the patient a bit.

- A patient in the out-patient lab does not speak English well. Eva uses diagrams to help explain how to provide a urine sample.

- Eva has a quick chat with a lab assistant who is arriving for the night shift. Eva lets her know about two patients who cannot have their blood collected for the next 24 hours.

- A student lab assistant is in the lab on practicum. Eva shows her around the lab and explains lab procedures and policies.

- Eva spends time on the phone confirming details with doctors about their test requisitions.

- Eva is entering data from test requisitions into the computer. A new doctor on staff asks Eva about test results. He wants to know how long it usually takes to get results when samples are shipped out to other labs.

Lab assistants communicate with many people.

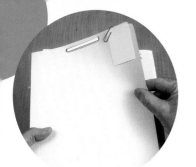

Essential Skill: Document Use

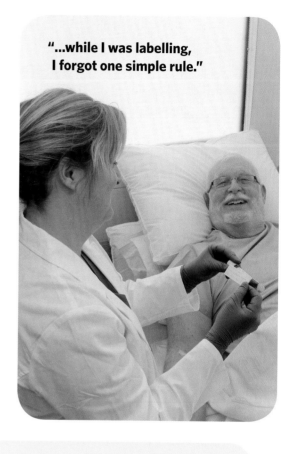

"...while I was labelling, I forgot one simple rule."

Eva learns how important it is to be accurate when working with documents.

Eva's story

When I take a blood sample from a patient, I have to label the sample right there, before I leave the room. All I have to do is peel the label off a roll of labels and stick it on to the tube that has the patient's blood in it. Should be easy, right? Well, one time while I was labelling, I forgot one simple rule.

It turned out one label didn't have the patient's last name on it, but I didn't catch it. I don't know. The patient, who liked to flirt, probably distracted me. I always, always double-check the information on labels before I stick them on the tubes. The sample was packed and sent to another lab for testing. Then that lab called our lab to say they couldn't use the sample because the label only had the patient's first name on it. A lot of people have the same first name, so the lab couldn't confirm the patient's identity. Of course, it was easy to look up the patient's last name at our end, but rules are rules. If a patient's full name isn't on the label, the sample can't be used for tests.

And to make things worse, that patient had been discharged and had to make a trip back to the hospital's out-patient lab just for a blood test. Boy! So much time and energy wasted because of not focusing on one "little" rule—double-check, double-check, double-check.

Another key essential skill for lab assistants is using documents. Eva learned through experience how important it is to be accurate when working with any kind of document—in this case, labels. She learned that a few seconds of double-checking can save a lot of time and energy later on.

Health care professionals use lab documents to make decisions about people's health and lives. Every document must be handled with care by every member of a lab team.

It's the law!

Lab records are legal documents that can be used in a court of law.

All in a day's work

- Eva fills in forms for blood samples that will be shipped to a special lab for testing.
- Eva helps a co-worker double-check a packing list for 90 urine specimens that need to be shipped out.
- Eva is collecting a blood sample from a young girl. The mother is at the girl's bedside. The girl jerks her arm and the needle slips out of the vein and pricks the mother's hand. Eva fills out an incident report.
- Eva has trouble collecting a blood sample from a patient. The patient has very tiny veins. Eva notes this fact on the sample collection list.
- Eva spends two hours entering test requisition data into a database.
- Eva fills in her online timesheet. She includes her break times and notes that she went to a training course one morning that week.

Lab assistants must be accurate when working with documents.

Lab assistants use online documents and databases.

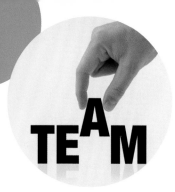

TE**A**M

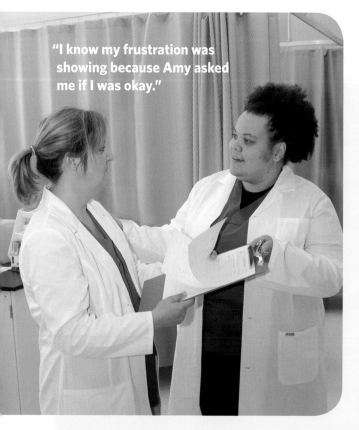

"I know my frustration was showing because Amy asked me if I was okay."

Eva gets a helping hand.

bathroom when I showed up, so I had to wait again. A couple of patients were just plain grumpy. Then a patient's husband stopped me in the hall. He started complaining to me about how his wife couldn't sleep the night before and that the nurses wouldn't give her something to sleep.

My head started to throb. I hadn't eaten anything for breakfast because I had slept in and didn't want to be late for work, and when I'm hungry, I get a headache. And then I'm irritable.

Eva's story

I was having a horrible day. Two lab assistants were off sick so that meant the rest of us had to pick up the slack. I had a lot of samples to collect that morning and it seemed every second patient had something going on. A doctor was talking to one of the patients so I had to wait for her to leave before I could draw blood. Then one patient was in the

I know my frustration was showing because Amy asked me if I was okay. I told Amy, my co-worker, that I was really behind schedule. Amy was already finished her collections and came to my rescue. She offered to do some of my collections, and I gratefully gave her one of my collection sheets. I was still behind schedule, but I felt better knowing I had support.

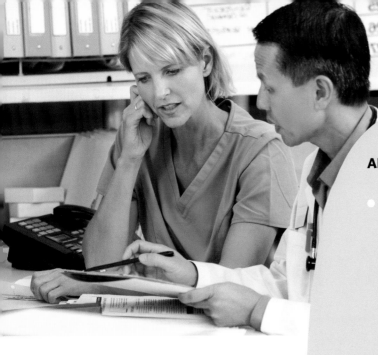

Lab assistants work with other members of the health care profession every day.

Being able to work with others is a key skill for lab assistants. "Others" for lab assistants includes a long list of people, from members of the lab team to health care professionals to patients.

Like Eva, all lab assistants are part of a team. The team may consist of three members or thirty members. Members of the team depend on one another for support. Support can mean working as a group to achieve a goal, giving advice, or sometimes acting as a leader. Working well together means that nobody on the team is afraid to offer help, or ask for it.

All in a day's work

- Eva attends the morning meeting. The head nurse thanks the staff, who have been working extra hard during the start of the flu season. She says the staff deserve to do something fun. Eva offers to take the lead in organizing a potluck.

- Eva has lunch with a co-worker who is new on the team. The co-worker tells Eva that he is nervous drawing blood from patients. Eva advises him that if he focuses on procedure, everything else will fall into place.

- The head nurse calls a quick meeting and explains a change in procedure. A co-worker passes on the information to Eva, who was not able to attend the meeting.

- A co-worker lost his home to a fire. The members of Eva's lab team get together and brainstorm ways to raise money for their co-worker.

Lab assistants work together for the well-being of patients and for the well-being of one another.

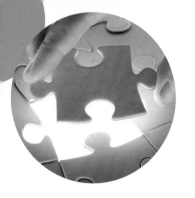

Essential Skill: Problem-Solving

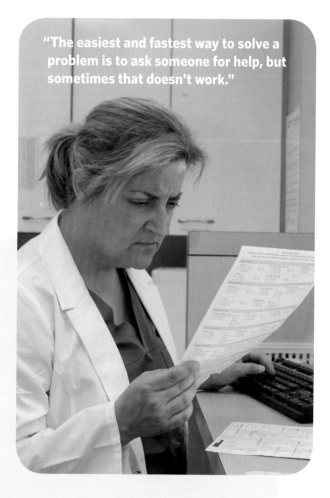

"The easiest and fastest way to solve a problem is to ask someone for help, but sometimes that doesn't work."

Eva has to figure out a doctor's secret code.

Eva's story

Part of my job is to enter the data from test requisitions into an online database. The tests are all listed on the requisition forms so doctors just have to check boxes, but some doctors handwrite the tests they want in the margins of the requisition forms. I don't know why they do that. It's faster to check off boxes.

I was entering requisition data one day and saw a handwritten code I'd never seen before. The easiest and fastest way to solve a problem is to ask someone for help, but sometimes that doesn't work. No one in the lab could figure out what test the doctor wanted.

I went into the files and found another requisition by the same doctor. It had the same "secret"

code on it. Then I checked our online database to see how the code had been entered into our system. It seemed the doctor wanted an HIV test done. Just to make sure, I phoned the doctor's office. His admin assistant said, "Yeah, that's just the way he writes it."

Next time I see that secret code, I'll know what it means.

Being able to solve problems is an essential skill for everyone. Lab assistants develop the skills to solve problems through training and experience. They learn to identify problems and take steps to solve them.

One strategy that Eva used to try to solve her problem was asking for help from others. When asking for help didn't work, Eva became creative and figured out another way to solve the problem.

In some cases, lab assistants can solve problems on their own. In other cases, they need to ask for support from others. The work lab assistants do affects people's lives and health, so they should never hesitate to ask questions or ask for help when in doubt.

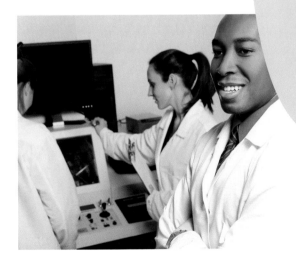

All in a day's work

- Eva is about to do a pregnancy test on a urine sample. She notices the patient's name is Alex Davies. Eva contacts the doctor who ordered the test. The doctor confirms that Alex Davies is female, so Eva does the test.

- A patient grumbles at Eva and refuses to let her collect a sample of blood. Eva makes a note on the blood collection schedule. Eva tries again later that morning. The patient is in better spirits and Eva is able to collect the sample.

- The printer that prints out labels for specimen bottles is not working. Eva informs the tech department. Eva fills in labels by hand until the printer is fixed.

- Eva notices that the label on a **bone marrow** specimen does not have a medical record number on it. Eva knows that bone marrow specimens cannot be collected again easily. She asks the lab manager what to do.

Lab assistants learn when to solve problems on their own and when to ask for help

Members of a lab team work together to solve problems.

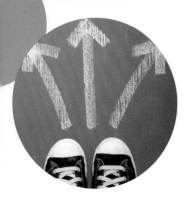

Essential Skill: Decision-Making

Eva makes a decision that upsets a patient.

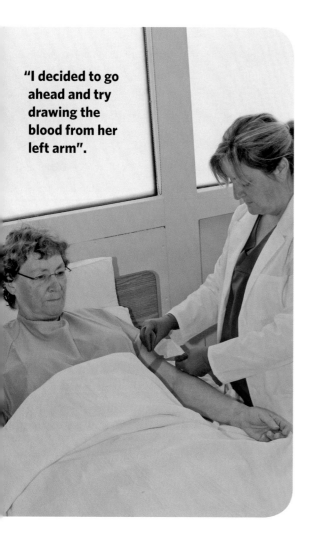

"I decided to go ahead and try drawing the blood from her left arm".

Eva's story

I was with Mrs. Leno, a patient, preparing to collect her blood. Mrs. Leno extended her right arm, ready to have her blood taken. That arm was bruised from having daily blood samples collected, so I said that I would collect the sample from her left arm. Mrs. Leno insisted that I collect the blood from her right arm. She told me that the other lab assistants always collected blood from that arm. She said that one lab assistant had tried to draw blood from her left arm but couldn't do it. Then another lab assistant tried, and she couldn't find a good vein either.

I examined the veins in Mrs. Leno's left arm. The veins were certainly deeper in that arm than in her right arm, but I was confident that I could get the sample. I asked Mrs. Leno to trust me. She wasn't happy and started grumbling at me, but I decided to go ahead and try drawing the blood from her left arm. And it worked. First poke.

I smiled at Mrs. Leno. She still looked grumpy. She said, "Now I'll have bruises on both arms."

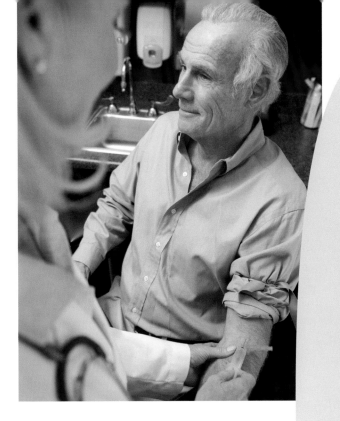

Lab assistants need to decide how to approach patients and clients.

Like solving problems, making decisions is a skill people use every day. Eva had to decide whether or not to take a blood sample from Mrs. Leno's left arm. She could have prevented upsetting Mrs. Leno by taking the sample from her right arm. But Eva knew that it would be more comfortable for Mrs. Leno if she took the sample from her left arm. Eva learned that sometimes decisions do not make everyone happy.

Lab assistants make many decisions in a day—some big, some small. The important thing is that they make decisions based on patients' well-being.

All in a day's work

- Eva has to collect a blood sample from a new patient. The patient is an older man. He is quite serious and does not talk much. Eva decides not to make cheery chitchat with this patient. It would probably annoy him. Eva just gets down to business.

- Eva needs to collect blood for the first time from a patient. She looks at the size of the veins in the patient's arm. She determines how close the veins are to the surface of the arm. She decides which needle to use to draw blood.

- Eva is supposed to collect a blood sample from a patient after every meal. The patient has eaten very little for lunch. Eva is not sure if the patient has eaten enough. She decides to ask the patient's nurse whether or not she should collect the blood sample from the patient.

- Eva is working in the emergency room. In the late afternoon, there is some downtime. No new patients have arrived in emergency. Eva decides to use the downtime to read a manual on first aid. There's always something new to learn.

Lab assistants have to decide when to make a decision and when to ask for help.

45

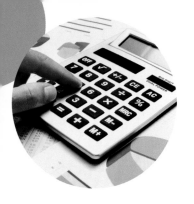

Essential Skill: Numeracy

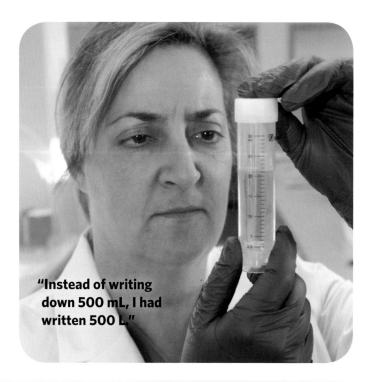

Eva learns a lesson about doing tasks with numbers.

"Instead of writing down 500 mL, I had written 500 L."

Eva's story

I was working in the lab one afternoon. It had been a pretty hectic day and I was trying to finish everything I needed to get done before going home. One thing I still had to do was measure how much urine was in some samples.

Things were moving along pretty well. I was working fast but carefully. I was in the middle of measuring one sample when I heard a co-worker curse out loud. She had spilled a whole container of blue dye on the floor. It was a real mess. I quickly finished measuring and wrote down how much urine was in the sample. Then I helped my co-worker clean up the dye. After that, I went back to measuring the samples.

The lab manager was reading the last measurement I had written down. He said maybe I should measure that sample again. I looked at what I had written and started to laugh. I had written that the sample contained 500 litres of urine. Wow! That was enough urine to fill the gas tanks of a dozen cars! Instead of writing down 500 mL, I had written 500 L. The missing *m* sure made a difference.

Lab assistants need to add, subtract, multiply, and divide numbers. They need to round off numbers and estimate. They work with fractions, decimals, and **ratios**. Lab assistants also need to measure things such as the volume, size, and weight of samples.

In smaller clinics, lab assistants may need to work with cash and credit card payments. They may need to estimate wait times for patients or estimate numbers of items when they check inventory.

Eva is quite comfortable working with numbers. However, Eva was reminded that having excellent numeracy skills is not enough. She also has to stay focused when working with numbers.

All in a day's work

- Eva counts how many samples were collected during a shift. Then she makes sure the count matches the total number of samples that were collected from the wards.

- Eva estimates how much cleaning fluid she needs to add to water to clean some lab equipment.

- The lab technologist shows Eva how to mix a solution using three liquids in a ratio of 1:3:2.

- Eva measures out 25 mL specimens of urine into separate tubes.

Working with numbers is an important part of a lab assistant's workday.

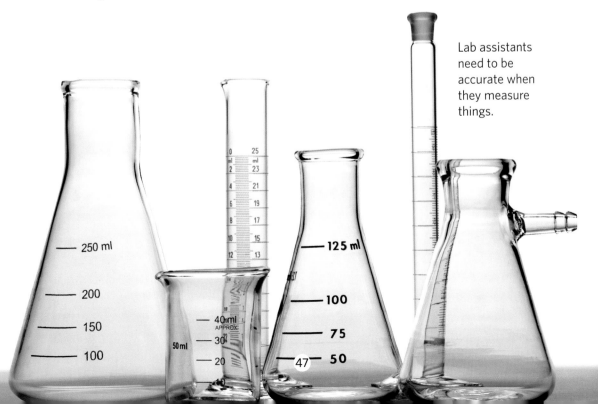

Lab assistants need to be accurate when they measure things.

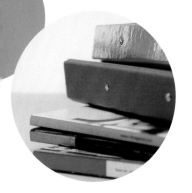

Essential Skill: Reading

Eva reads her way
out of a mess.

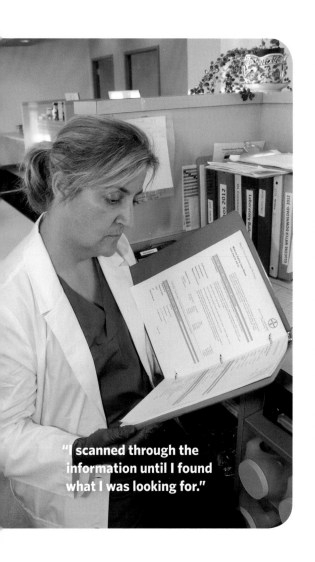

"I scanned through the information until I found what I was looking for."

Eva's story

I was in the stockroom getting something for a lab technologist. I pushed a bottle to one side to get at what I wanted, but I pushed it too far. The bottle went crashing to the floor. Some kind of liquid splashed out all over the floor. I didn't know what the liquid was, so I couldn't clean it up. It could have been **toxic** or **corrosive**. I had no idea.

I looked at a similar bottle on the shelf and got the name of the liquid. Then I got the MSDS manual. MSDS stands for Material Safety Data Sheet. The sheet tells us everything we need to know about using chemicals safely. I scanned through the information until I found what I was looking for: how toxic the liquid might be and how to clean it up.

I followed the steps in the MSDS for cleaning the liquid up and then told the lab tech what had happened. I filled in an incident report.

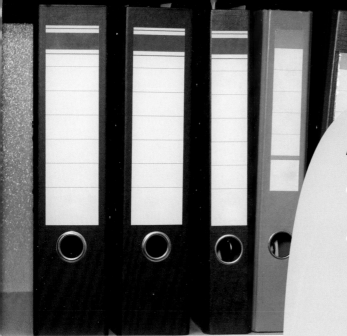

Lab assistants need to read a lot of procedure manuals.

Reading is an essential skill for lab assistants. Lab assistants read documents and forms every day. They also read logbooks and manuals as well as memos and notes.

Like Eva, lab assistants need strong reading skills to make sure that they can work safely and independently.

All in a day's work

- Eva reads a memo about a change in how to dispose of broken glass.

- Eva reads the lab logbook. A note in the logbook tells her that a piece of equipment is not working. The note also says that a technician was called and would arrive before noon.

- Eva needs to write a test on safety in the lab to keep her certification. She finds time to study one unit in the safety manual.

- A co-worker leaves a note for Eva. The note asks Eva to check whether some samples that the lab manager has been waiting for have arrived.

- Eva is taking a course in how to prepare biohazardous materials for shipping. She reads over some handouts.

- During her break, Eva reads something interesting in the hospital's monthly newsletter. The local university is asking for volunteers to be in a research study. The study is looking at how peas and beans affect levels of cholesterol. Eva thinks she might sign up as a volunteer for the study.

Reading helps lab assistants work safely and make independent decisions.

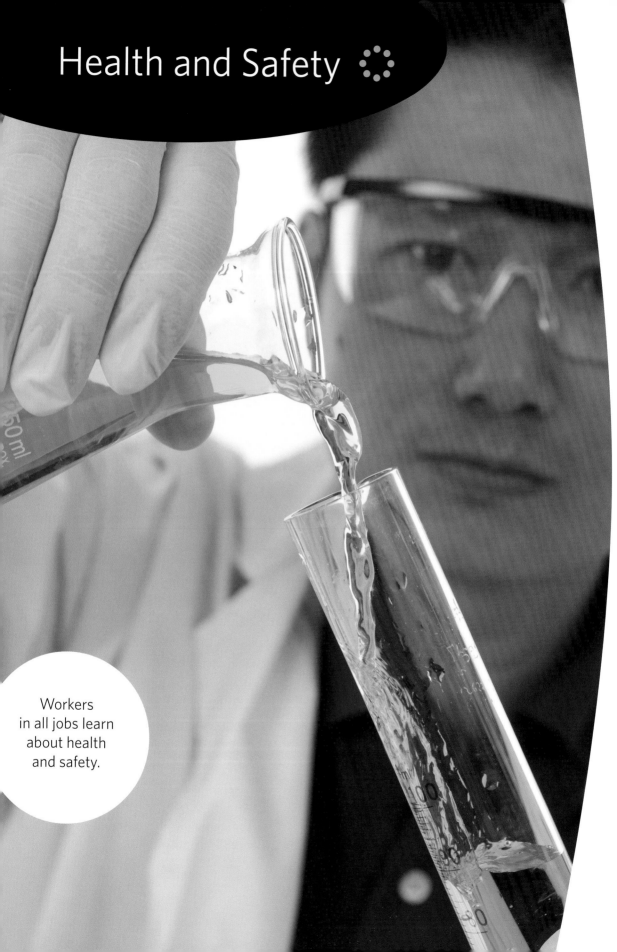

Health and Safety

Workers in all jobs learn about health and safety.

Health and Safety

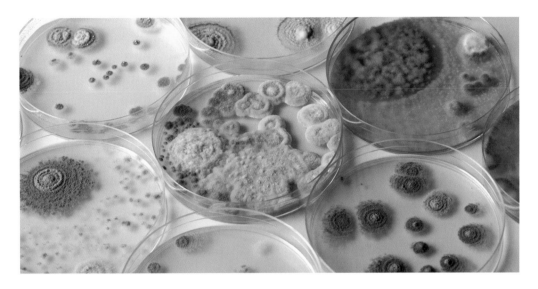

Lab assistants learn to work safely with micro-organisms, such as bacteria.

Roy was removing a glass tube from a cold container. The tube held a sample of blood. All of a sudden, the tube shattered. Some of the blood splashed on Roy's face.

Roy went to the eyewash station. He removed his goggles and latex gloves. He threw the gloves in a waste bin marked biohazards. He put on a new pair of gloves. He started to splash warm water on his face. He rinsed his face for 15 minutes. Then Roy told the lab supervisor what had happened and filled in an incident report.

Lab assistants work with biohazards like tissue, blood, and body fluids and solids. Biohazards contain many kinds of **micro-organisms**. Micro-organisms may cause infection if they touch the skin or enter the body through a cut or wound. Micro-organisms can also enter the body through contact with the eyes, nose, and lips. Some micro-organisms, like certain bacteria and viruses, can escape into the air and may be breathed in.

Lab assistants learn to work safely with biohazards, such as blood.

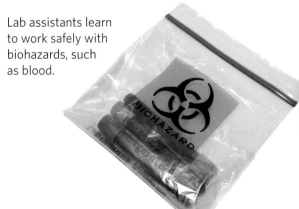

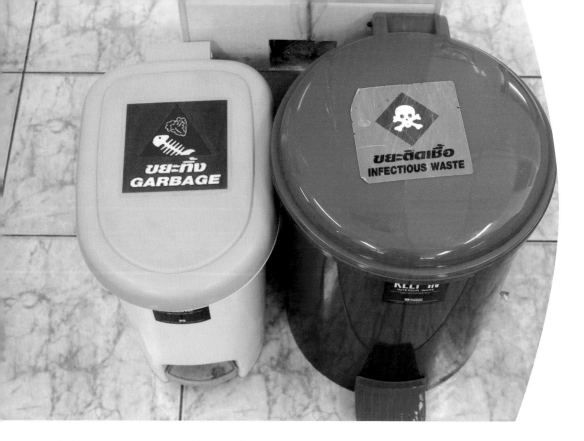

Lab assistants are trained how to dispose of hazardous materials.

Lab assistants are trained how to handle biohazards in a safe way. For example, they wear gloves at all times. They know when to wear safety goggles and masks. They are trained in how to store and dispose of biohazards. Lab assistants are also trained in how to prevent possible infection, as in Roy's case.

Workers in all jobs need to know about health and safety. For a lab assistant, health and safety means knowing how to work with **biological** materials. It also means being aware of chemical hazards and physical hazards.

Lab assistants learn how and when to wash their hands.

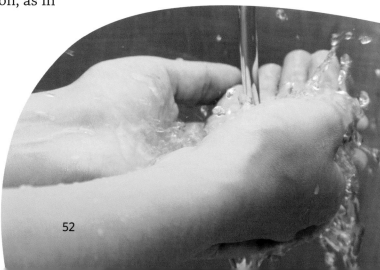

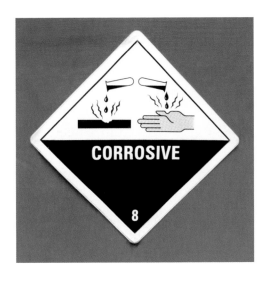

Lab assistants learn how to read warning symbols.

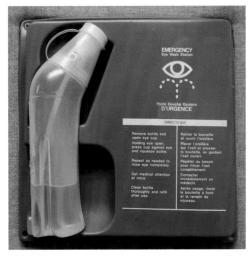

All labs have eyewash stations.

Chemical hazards

What is the most common chemical found in people's homes? The answer is bleach. Bleach is also used in labs. Lab assistants use bleach, and other chemicals, to clean instruments, work surfaces, equipment, and glassware.

Some lab assistants work with chemicals every day. They often use chemicals when preparing samples for testing. Some chemicals are dangerous to work with because they catch fire easily. Other chemicals are corrosive, which means they can cause severe burns if they come in contact with the skin. Still other chemicals give off toxic gases that can cause harm if they are breathed in. Some chemicals are safe and only become hazardous when they come in contact with other chemicals.

Lab assistants are careful when using chemicals in the workplace. Lab assistants are trained in how to use chemicals, store chemicals, and dispose of chemicals. They learn what to do in the case of chemical spills and exposure to chemical gases.

hazard: a source of danger or risk that can cause illness or injuries to the body, such as bleeding from cuts or loss of hearing and vision; *hazardous* means dangerous.

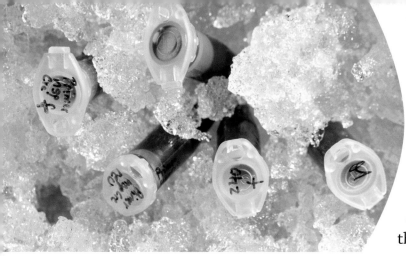

Lab assistants pack samples in dry ice.

Physical hazards

Ouch! A paper cut is minor, but it can really hurt. After getting a few paper cuts, people probably adjust how they handle paper. In other words, they learn how to work with the physical hazard—paper.

A lab is home to many physical hazards. For example, dry ice is a hazard. Dry ice is so cold it freezes skin and tissue on contact. Lab assistants may be asked to pack blood samples in dry ice for transport.

Lab assistants work with needles and syringes. They need to know how to use needles safely and how to dispose of used needles and syringes. Medical groups and employers work hard to make sure that lab assistants work in safe environments, where the chance of being hurt with needles remains very low.

Sometimes lab assistants need to carry or move cylinders full of gas that is under high pressure. Lab assistants may work around high levels of electrical currents. Or they may work near materials that are **carcinogenic**. For example, formaldehyde is a gas that is used in labs. It is used to preserve biological samples such as tissue samples. Formaldehyde is carcinogenic.

Lab assistants work with health and safety hazards every day. However, serious accidents in a lab are rare. All members of a lab team are trained in how to work safely in areas that have physical hazards. All members of a lab team pay strict attention to lab rules at all times.

It's the law!

Employers must provide safe and healthy work sites. For example, they must equip every work site with a safe system of air vents.

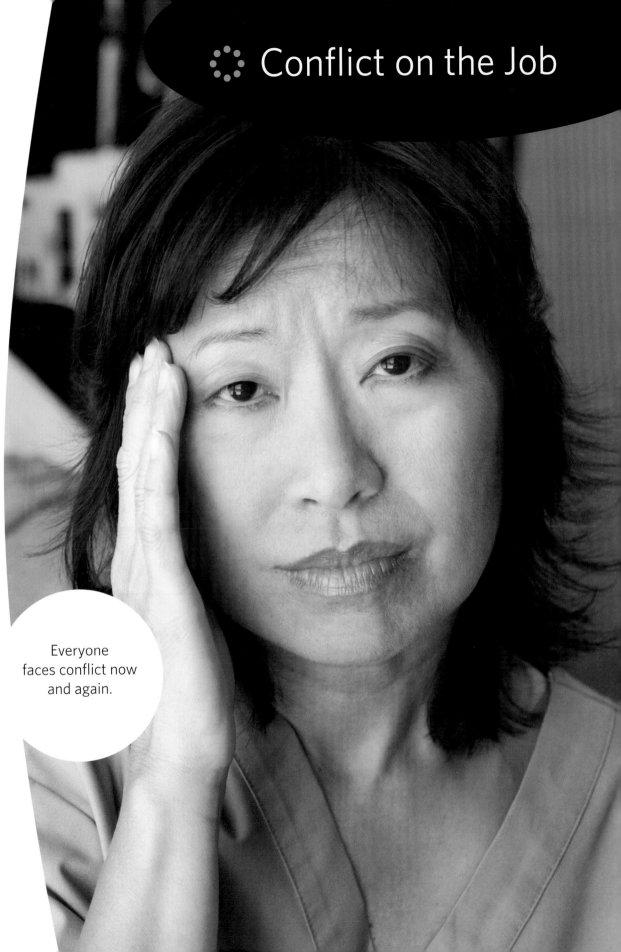

Conflict on the Job

Everyone faces conflict now and again.

Conflict on the Job

When was the last time you disagreed with someone? When was the last time you felt tense in a relationship or wondered why someone was acting strange?

Nobody is perfect. And sometimes, even people we like can frustrate us. Everyone faces **conflict** with family and friends now and again. And everyone faces conflict on the job now and again.

Lab assistants work in a range of work settings, which means they work with a range of people.

Some lab assistants work with only two or three other people on a daily basis. Others may have contact with dozens of people, from patients to doctors to co-workers. Whatever the work setting, conflict may occur. People have unique personalities. They bring their values and opinions to the workplace. They all have ideas of *what* should be done and *how* it should be done. It is not surprising, then, that most lab assistants experience some conflict on the job.

Conflict with others

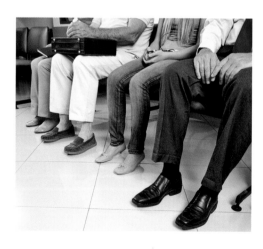

"My co-worker is so chatty with the clients, even when we have a waiting room full of people waiting to get their tests done. Drives me crazy."

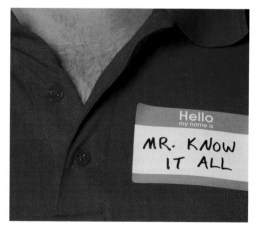

Hello
my name is
MR. KNOW
IT ALL

"I'm in charge of a student who's doing his practicum in our lab. He doesn't listen! He thinks he knows everything. It's so annoying."

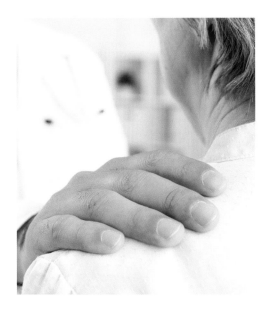

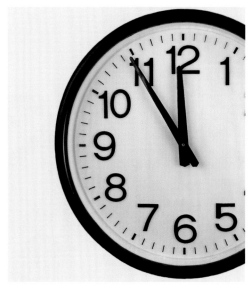

"One lab assistant always touches my arm or puts his hand on my shoulder when we talk. I'm not a touchy person. He does it to everyone. Maybe it's a cultural thing."

"We're usually rushed for time to get test results out by noon. But still, I find it annoying when co-workers forget that clients are people. They're not cattle to be pushed through a gate."

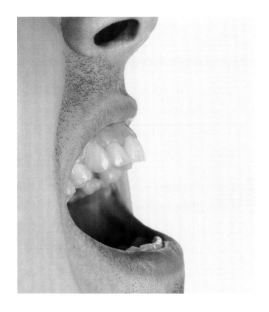

Lab assistants learn how to recognize conflict and work with others to end conflict.

"Some days it seems the clients are so grouchy. No one likes going for tests, right? But still, sometimes I just want to scream. But I can't. That wouldn't be professional."

Self-conflict

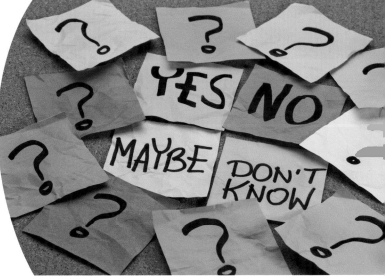

Tracy works at a clinic and is good at her job. Although she has been at the clinic for only a few months, she has won the respect of the other members on the lab team.

One day, Tracy's favourite aunt, Aunt Jane, fell ill. The illness started with a severe fever. After that, Jane got headaches, was dizzy all the time, and had trouble keeping her balance. Jane's doctor requisitioned a series of tests.

Tracy's mother was concerned about her sister's health. Tracy's mother and Jane were more than sisters; they were best friends. Tracy's mother knew that Jane's tests were being carried out at the clinic where Tracy worked. Tracy's mother asked her to find out the results of Jane's tests. Tracy explained that she couldn't do that. She explained that she

didn't see the results of the tests. Tracy's mother told her to ask the lab technologists about the results. Tracy said she couldn't do that. She told her mother that she would have to be patient and wait until the doctor told Jane the results.

Tracy's mother asked Tracy about the results every day for days on end, saying that Tracy could find out about the results if she really wanted to. Tracy's mother became angry. She accused Tracy of not caring about her, or her Aunt Jane.

Tracy was in conflict with herself. She hated seeing her mother so upset. At the same time, she knew that she had no right to ask about her aunt's test results. And she knew if she did ask the lab technologist about her aunt's results, she would be asking the technologist to go against the **code of ethics**.

All lab assistants follow a code of ethics. The code of ethics helps lab assistants make decisions based on what is right and what is wrong. One principal point in the code of ethics is respect for patients' privacy. The code of ethics says that test results can only be released to the health care professionals who requisitioned the tests. Tracy would have to be strong enough to stand up to her mother's anger.

Lab assistants are not alone when dealing with conflict. They can turn to friends and family for help and advice. They can keep in touch with someone who acts as their mentor, or advisor. A mentor can be a teacher or a member of a lab team with many years of work experience.

Lab assistants can also join groups for support. They can join a professional group, or they can form a support group with co-workers or by keeping in touch with a few trusted classmates.

Dealing with conflict is never easy in any job, whether it is self-conflict or conflict with others. If conflict goes on for a long time, it can lead to stress. In a healthy workplace, all members of a lab team work together to prevent conflict.

Glossary

bacteria: a medical name for germs.

beaker: a glass container shaped like a tube and used for science experiments.

biohazard: a danger to health that comes from biological work. Example: Blood is a biohazard because it might carry harmful micro-organisms.

biological: having to do with living things. Example: Harmful germs are used in biological weapons.

blood transfusion: the injection of blood from a healthy person into a patient who needs it.

bone marrow: the soft, fatty material in bones that is used to form blood cells.

carcinogenic: producing cancer. Example: Tobacco smoke is carcinogenic.

cholera: a disease of the small intestine, which is caused by a type of bacteria.

cholesterol: a material found in human tissue and blood that causes the walls of arteries to thicken and harden.

code of ethics: rules about how to act based on what is right and what is wrong.

conflict: when what one person wants or needs does not match what another person wants or needs.

corrosive: causing something to wear away, usually by chemical action. Example: Drain cleaners contain corrosive chemicals so that they can clear out clogged pipes.

dementia: a group of illnesses that affect memory, behaviour, learning, and communication.

ECG: short term for electrocardiogram; a heart test.

flask: a glass container with a narrow neck used in chemistry.

microbiology: the study of tiny living things, like bacteria.

micro-organism: a living thing that can only be seen through a microscope. Examples: bacteria, viruses.

pipette: a thin tube used for measuring and transferring small amounts of liquid.

plasma: a clear liquid in the blood.

ratio: how two things are related in terms of size, amount, or number. Example: A pail is filled with 10 cups of liquid. The liquid is made up of bleach and water. The ratio of bleach to water is 9 to 1. That means there are 9 cups of bleach and 1 cup of water in the pail.

saliva: the liquid that your mouth produces; often called spit.

slide: a small, thin piece of glass that holds objects to be examined under a microscope. Example: The lab assistant put a thin slice of tissue on the slide.

specimen: part of a sample.

stool: feces.

tissue: the material that makes up parts of the body. Examples: muscle tissue, brain tissue, lung tissue.

toxic: poisonous.

toxin: a poison caused by a living thing.

typhoid: a severe fever, which is caused by a type of bacteria.

Photo credits